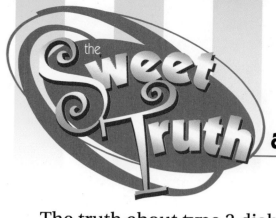

the Sweet Truth about managing type 2 diabetes

The truth about type 2 diabetes is that you will have it for the rest of your life. So, the more you learn about living with it, the better off you will be. Why? Because, learning about your diabetes can help you control it. And when your diabetes is under control you can lead a happy, healthy and active life.

Whether you have just found out you have diabetes or have had it for some time, this book will help you learn:

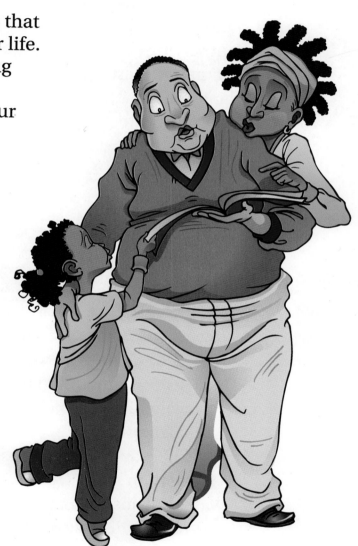

- what type 2 diabetes is
- how it is treated
- how you can prevent problems
- your part in managing it

Share this book with your family. Talk with them about your diabetes and how you need to control your blood glucose levels. Work with your family and your health care team to make living with diabetes a little easier.

1

Table of contents

What type 2 diabetes means

Cells are building blocks of the body. They need energy to do their job. This **energy comes from food.**

Some foods (carbohydrates) are quickly broken down into sugar (glucose). Then **glucose** flows through the blood and into your cells. This **gives you the energy you need** each day.

When you have diabetes, your body can't use the energy it gets from food. **There is a problem with** a hormone made by your pancreas called **insulin.**

Glucose cannot get into your cells without insulin helping it. So, glucose stays in your blood and builds up.

Over time, too much glucose in the blood can cause problems with your eyes, kidneys, blood vessels, nerves, skin and feet (see pages 63-74).

Examples of carbohydrates

(car-bo-hi-drates)

Fruits
Starchy Vegetables
Rice
Cereal
Bread
Pasta
Dry Beans

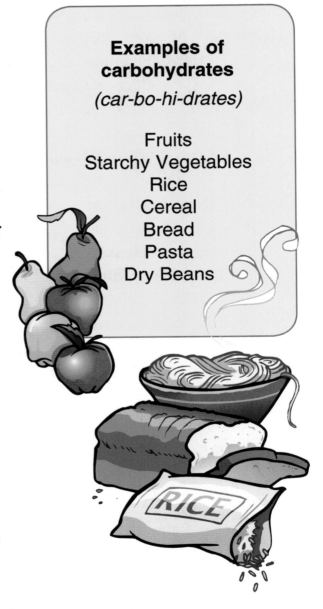

With type 2 diabetes, the problem is either that:

- your body does not make enough insulin
  <u>or</u>
- your body cannot use the insulin that it does make

When your body cannot use the insulin it makes, it is called **insulin resistance.** The insulin just does not work right. Overweight people often have problems with this.

This may be due to:

- **problems in the cells** where the insulin is working

- **medicines** (like steroids) that block insulin from working and raise blood glucose

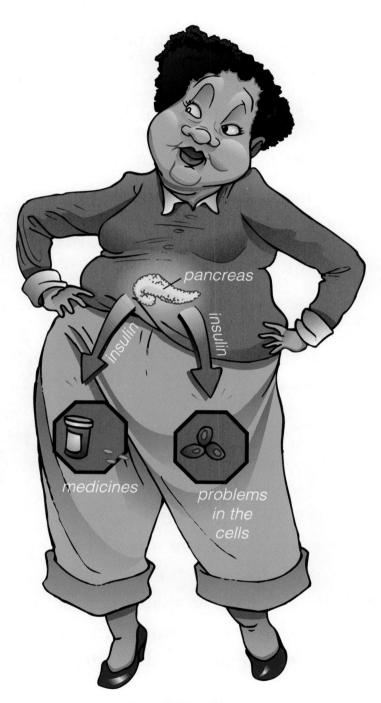

type 2 diabetes
insulin resistance

You may wonder what the big deal is about glucose. Well, for one thing, you cannot live without it. Your body needs glucose to:

- give you energy
- keep your brain, heart, liver and kidneys working
- help in nerve and muscle function

But when glucose cannot get into your cells it stays in your blood. It then spills over into your urine and is passed out of your body. When this happens **you may not have any symptoms** at all or you may:

- be tired and weak a lot
- have headaches, blurred vision or numbness (loss of feeling) in your hands, lower legs and feet
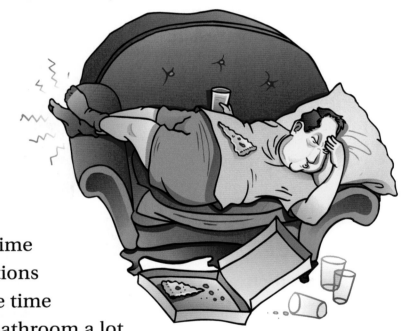
- always be thirsty
- be hungry all the time
- have a lot of infections
- feel nervous all the time
- have to go to the bathroom a lot
- not heal as fast as you normally would
- have itchy or dry skin

Type 2 is the most common type of diabetes. Some people call it "adult-onset diabetes." It often affects adults over age 30 who have a family history of diabetes, are overweight and do not exercise*. However, as many as 45% of children who are newly diagnosed with diabetes have type 2. This is because more children today are overweight and less active.

Type 2 diabetes can sometimes be controlled without having to take insulin. Some people can manage their glucose by controlling how many carbohydrates they eat and by exercising.

But, for those who cannot manage it with diet and exercise, oral medicines (pills), insulin or both may be needed.

Note:
If anyone in your family is overweight, it might be a good idea to have them check their blood glucose levels for early detection.

* *Native Americans, Hispanics, African Americans, Asians and Pacific Islanders are also at increased risk.*

How it is managed

Your goal is to get your blood **glucose level as normal as possible** (70-130 mg/dl before meals and less than 180 mg/dl 2 hours after a meal)* and keep it there.

Doing this involves:

- healthy meal planning
- exercising
- taking insulin and/or oral medicines
- blood glucose monitoring
- losing weight
- reducing stress

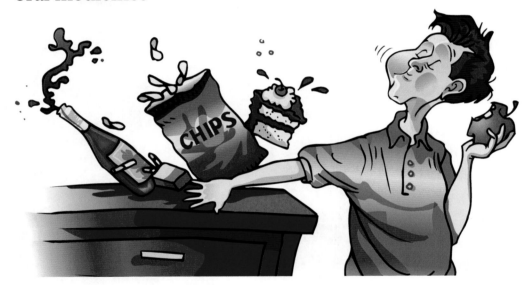

This might seem like a lot to do. But, if you make managing your diabetes part of your daily routine, it will be easier.

The steps you take in managing your diabetes are just like other things you do every day (like brushing your teeth). And, you can still live a "normal" life and do the things you want to do. And don't forget you are not alone. Your health care team is there to help you with each step you take.

* Your range may be different. Talk with your doctor about this.

Healthy Meal Planning

Food is the fuel for your body. **Meal planning** helps you get the right amount of "fuel" each day. How much is needed **varies from person to person**. How active you are, how much energy you need and your weight all have a part in how much food you need.

A healthy meal plan:

- gives you **healthy and balanced meals**
- gives you the **same amount of food** each day
- **spreads out what you eat** over the course of a day
- allows you to **enjoy the foods you prefer** to eat
- is flexible and **offers** you **choices**

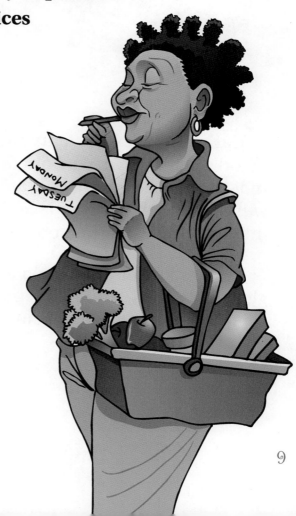

Your body may still make some insulin. So, you may not need to inject insulin or take pills for diabetes, as long as you eat a healthy diet. And a weight loss of 5-10 pounds can help, too (if you need to lose weight).

You don't have to go on a strange diet because you have diabetes. You just need to follow a healthy meal plan. That's the same for everyone—those who have diabetes and those who don't.

A word about food

All foods are made up of carbohydrates, proteins, fats, vitamins, minerals, water and fiber. So, your meal plan uses everyday foods. There are no "special," "forbidden" or "bad" foods.

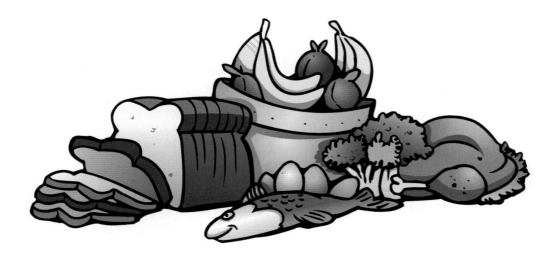

Carbohydrates, proteins and fat all affect your blood glucose. But, **carbohydrates affect it the most.** Almost all carbohydrates turn into glucose within 1½ hours after you eat them. Some turn into glucose faster than others.

It takes longer for protein to be turned into glucose (about 2½ hours). And, fat is turned into triglycerides (fatty acids) and stored for use as energy later.

Carbohydrates are the **main sources of fuel** for your body. They may be:

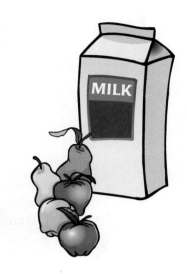

- Sugars (they turn into glucose the fastest)
- Starches (they take longer to turn into glucose)

We think about sugar as only table sugar. But, **syrup, honey, molasses,** fructose (in **fruits**) and lactose (in **milk**) **are also forms of sugar.**

The major sources of **starches** are:

- **grains**—bread, rice and pasta
- **vegetables**—potatoes and beans

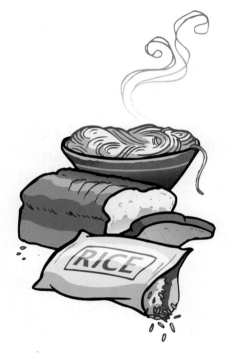

Grains and vegetables tend to have more vitamins, minerals, water and fiber, and they tend to be low in fat. "Sugary" foods, as a rule, do not have these other nutrients and they tend to have more fat. So, starches are better in helping you control your weight.

There are also non-starchy vegetables. They contain about ⅓ of the carbohydrates that starchy vegetables contain. These include green leafy vegetables (broccoli, greens, spinach, etc.) and brightly colored vegetables (yellow squash, carrots, zucchini, beets, etc.).

Protein is used to build muscles, organs, hormones and enzymes. Protein is mainly found in:

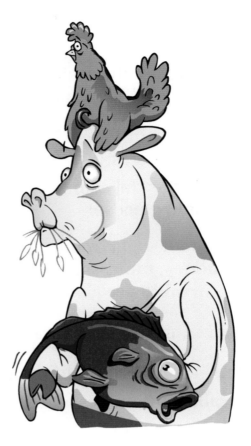

- meat
- poultry
- fish
- dairy products
- eggs
- soy beans
- tofu and other soy products

Fat helps:

- keep your skin and hair healthy
- carry vitamins through your intestinal tract and bloodstream
- control your blood cholesterol levels

Fats contain about twice the number of calories as carbohydrates and proteins. Any excess calories you eat are stored as body fat. So, eating too much of any type of fat can lead to being overweight or obese—a risk factor for heart disease.

When you exercise, your body uses this excess up slowly. After about 30 minutes of aerobic exercising, like brisk walking or riding a bicycle, your body starts to get its energy more from fats than from carbohydrates.

These are the main types of fats:

- **Saturated fats** come mainly from animal foods: meats, poultry and whole-milk dairy products. But some saturated fats come from plants: coconut oil, palm oil and palm kernel oil. Saturated fats **raise blood cholesterol levels.**

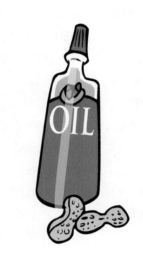

- **Polyunsaturated fats** come mainly from plant oils (corn, safflower and sesame oils) and walnuts. These fats can **help in reducing blood cholesterol levels.**

- **Monounsaturated fats** also come mainly from plant oils (canola, peanut and olive), olives and nuts (except walnuts). These fats can **help in lowering blood cholesterol levels,** also.

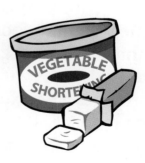

- **Trans fats** are made when vegetable oils are hydrogenated (hydrogen is added) so that they are solid at room temperature. Margarines, vegetable shortenings and food items that contain these are examples of trans fats. These fats **raise LDL ("bad") cholesterol and lower HDL ("good") cholesterol levels.**

Vitamins help your body make new tissue including teeth, bones and blood. They help regulate various functions within your cells, even though only small amounts are needed.

Minerals are needed to regulate the chemical balance between cells and **to keep your nerve functions healthy**. Your body needs more of some minerals than others.

Fiber comes from plants. One type of fiber (found mostly in wheat) helps prevent constipation. Another type of fiber is found in vegetables, fruits, beans, barley, oats and oat bran. This type of fiber helps lower your blood cholesterol. Lowering cholesterol helps reduce your risk of heart disease. Fiber is filling so you think you are full, yet it contains little fat. Because of this, fiber can help in controlling your weight.

Water makes up a very large part of the weight in food. It is needed by all the cells and organs in your body and your body needs a lot of it for good health. It provides a way for all chemicals in your body to react. It helps your blood circulate and your body remove waste. Water is a lubricant and it plays a big part in helping to control your body's temperature.

Counting carbohydrates

Carbohydrate (carb) counting is a way of figuring out how many grams of carbs you can eat at meals and snacks. You do this because carbs have the biggest effect on your blood glucose. All calories are turned into glucose, but not as fast as those from carbs.

As a rule, you can eat about half of your calories in carbohydrates. So if you can eat 1,600 calories a day, 800 of them can be carbs. There are 4 calories in each gram of carbohydrate. So, you can have about 200 grams each day (800 ÷ 4 = 200). The idea in counting carbs is to **spread those grams out over the course of a day.**

You need energy all day. Think about what would happen to your blood glucose and your energy level if you eat all your carbs at one meal. Your blood glucose would go very high, but after 1-1 ½ hours you would be hungry again because most of the fuel is gone.

This is where proteins come into play. They stay with you longer to give you that energy later on.

When you know how to count carbs, it is easier to plan your meals and snacks. Since **most of the carbs you eat come from starches, fruits, milk or non-starchy vegetables,** those are the foods you focus on.

Here are the approximate number of **grams (g) of carbs in 1 serving** of each food group:

Food Items (1 serving)	Carbs
Starches	15 g
Fruits	15 g
Milk products	12–15 g
Non-starchy vegetables	5 g
Meats and fats	0 g

You might think of 1 serving as 1 carb choice. If you can have 200 grams of carbs during the day, and each serving or choice counts as 15 grams, then throughout your day you can have 13 carb choices (200 ÷ 15 = 13.3).

Looking at the chart above, however, if you choose more non-starchy vegetables that only have 5 grams of carbs, you can eat 3 of them as 1 serving. And, you will still be following your meal plan.

About servings

The number of servings you can have of each food group depends on several factors. Your doctor, nurse, diabetes educator or registered dietitian can help you tailor your meal plan by looking at your:

- height
- weight
- activity level
- medicines (if any)
- likes and dislikes

All these together will help your dietitian decide how many calories you should have each day. And, based on that, you will learn the number of servings of each food group you can have. For example:

Number of servings you can have each day

Food Group	1600 calories	2000 calories	2400 calories	2800 calories
starches	6	8	11	12
milk	2	2	2	3
fruits	2	3	3	4
non-starchy vegetables	3	4	4	6
meat or meat substitutes	2	2	2	2
fats and sweets	3	4	5	5

What makes a serving?

Food Group	Examples	Carb Grams	Serving Size Examples
Starches			
	bread	15	1 slice bread, ½ English muffin, 1 small roll, a 6" tortilla
	grains	15	½ cup cooked grits, ⅓ cup cooked pasta, ⅓ cup cooked rice
	beans	15	½ cup cooked lima beans, ¼ cup baked beans
	starchy vegetables	15	⅓ cup
Fruits			
	fresh fruit	15	A 2" round apple, a 2¾" peach, 1 cup honeydew melon
	dried fruit	15	2½ dates, 2 Tbsp raisins, 4 apple (round slices)
	fruit juice	15	½ cup apple, orange or grapefruit juice, ⅓ cup cranberry juice
Vegetables			
	greens	5	½ cup cooked or 1 cup raw
	beets	5	½ cup cooked or 1 cup raw
	broccoli	5	½ cup cooked or 1 cup raw
	carrots	5	½ cup cooked or 1 cup raw
	asparagus	5	½ cup cooked or 1 cup raw
	vegetable juice	5	½ cup
Meats & meat substitutes			
	beef, pork chicken, fish	0	2-3 oz
	cheese	0	1 oz regular, ¼ cup cottage cheese
	eggs	0	1 egg, 3 egg whites
	nuts	0	6 dry roasted almonds, 1 Tbsp cashews, 20 small peanuts
Milk products			
	milk	12	1 cup skim milk, 1 cup 1% milk, ½ cup evaporated milk
	yogurt	12	8 oz plain yogurt
Fats & sweets			
	salad dressing	0	1 Tbsp regular
	mayonnaise	0	2 Tbsp
	butter	0	1 tsp
	bacon	0	1 slice
	heavy cream	0	1 Tbsp
	ice cream	15	½ cup ice cream, ¼ cup sherbet, ½ cup ice milk
	cake, cookies, pie	15	6 small vanilla wafers, 1 plain cake doughnut, a 3" cookie

Serving sizes

These quick reminders can help you get a feel for what a serving size looks like. With practice, you will be able to gauge them without measuring.

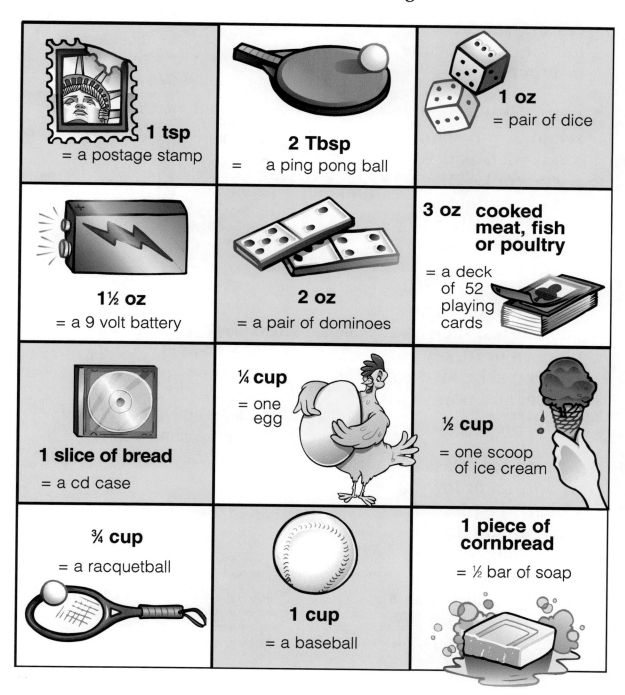

1 tsp = a postage stamp

2 Tbsp = a ping pong ball

1 oz = pair of dice

1½ oz = a 9 volt battery

2 oz = a pair of dominoes

3 oz cooked meat, fish or poultry = a deck of 52 playing cards

1 slice of bread = a cd case

¼ cup = one egg

½ cup = one scoop of ice cream

¾ cup = a racquetball

1 cup = a baseball

1 piece of cornbread = ½ bar of soap

Create your plate

1. In the largest section, add non-starchy vegetables such as carrots, spinach, lettuce, green beans or broccoli.

2. In one of the small sections, put starchy foods such as rice, pasta, cooked beans or peas, potatoes, corn or lima beans.

3. In the last small section, place your meat or meat substitutes, such as chicken or turkey without skin, lean cuts of beef and pork, fish or tofu.

4. Add an 8oz. glass of non-fat or low-fat milk and a piece of fruit. If you don't drink milk, you can add another small serving of carb, like a 6oz. container of light yogurt or a small roll.

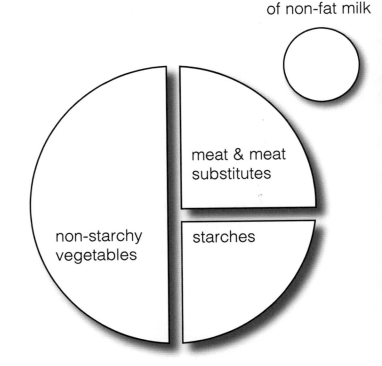

8 oz. glass of non-fat milk

meat & meat substitutes

non-starchy vegetables

starches

Reminder Note:

The more active you are, the more calories you need.

<u>AND</u>

The less active you are, the fewer calories you need.

I should eat _____ calories a day.

*Copyright 2013 American Diabetes Association
From http://www.diabetes.org
Reprinted with permission from the American
Diabetes Association*

Let's take a look at a food label

The serving size on the food label and the serving size on your meal plan may not be the same.

Note that one serving (½ cup) of this product is 2 servings (30g) of carbohydrates (1 carb serving=12-15g).

The **percentage** of daily value **is based on a 2,000 calorie a day diet**. This may or may not be right for your meal plan. As you learn more, you may have to adjust your meal plan based on the facts on food labels.

Look at the number of grams in each serving. Then, compare that to the number of grams in your meal plan.

For each meal, try to **eat no more than 5-10 g of fat and 45-60 g of carbohydrate*.** (For a snack, no more than 15 g of carbohydrate.) And, try to use products that have at least 2-3g of fiber in them.

Nutrition Facts

Serving Size ½ cup
Servings Per Container 5

Amount Per Serving

Calories 250   Calories from Fat 110

% Daily Value*

Total Fat 12g		**19%**
Saturated Fat 5g		**25%**
Trans Fat 4g		
Cholesterol 25 mg		**9%**
Sodium 650 mg		**28%**
Total Carbohydrate 30g		**10%**
Dietary Fiber 0g		**0%**
Sugars 5g		
Protein 5g		

Vitamin A 3%	•	Vitamin C 2%

* Percent Daily Values are based on a 2,000 calorie diet. Your daily values may be higher or lower depending on your calorie needs:

	Calories	2,000	2,500
Total Fat	Less than	65g	80g
Sat Fat	Less than	20g	25g
Cholesterol	Less than	300mg	300mg
Sodium	Less than	2,400mg	2,400mg
Total Carbohydrate		300g	375g
Dietary Fiber		25g	30g

1g Fat = 9 calories
1g Carbohydrates = 4 calories
1 g Protein = 4 calories

***Note:** These are general guidelines. Your meal plan may vary.*

A food diary

A **food diary** is a **record of what and when you eat and drink during a day.**

This diary can show the healthy foods you already eat and the foods you should eat less of—those high in fat, sweets or with hidden fats or salt, etc. It can also show:

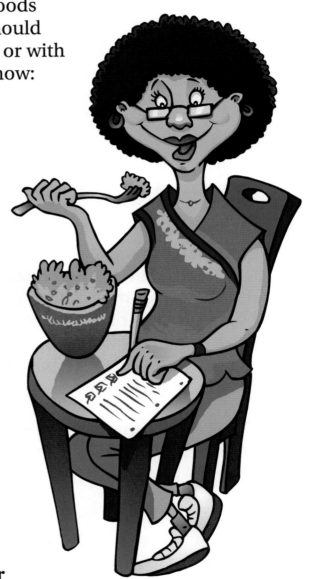

- serving sizes
- skipped meals
- snacks
- the kinds of foods you eat most
- your eating pattern

Keep your food diary for 3 or 4 days. Use 2 workdays and 1 weekend day (or your day off). List all foods eaten and how they are cooked. This will show your diabetes educator or dietitian what your food habits are and what changes may be needed. Then a meal plan can be made just for you.

Also **fill in your blood glucose levels before and after each meal or snack.** This can help you see how the foods you eat affect your blood glucose.

How to complete your food diary

Make extra copies of the food diary on the next page. You'll need one for each day. Then:

- in the **Food Items** column, list the name of each item you eat at each meal or snack and the time you eat it
- on the line with the name of the meal or snack, fill in **How** it is **Cooked**
- in the **Serving Size** column, fill in how much you eat
- fill in your **Blood Glucose Readings** for each meal (or snack)
- take each page with you to your next visit **(Your diabetes educator or dietitian will fill in the rest of the diary.)**

Here's how to do it:

Food Items	How Cooked	Serving Size	Blood Glucose Readings		
			before meals	1 hour after	2 hours after
Breakfast/ 7:13 am			107	170	135
egg	fried	1 egg			
bacon	microwaved	2 strips			
white bread	toasted	2 slices			
butter for toast		1 Tbsp			
black coffee		1 cup			
Lunch/ 12:15 pm			120	180	140
ham and cheese sandwich on rye with mustard only	pre-packaged meat/cheese	2 slices (rye bread) 1 oz cheese (1 slice American) 3 oz ham (3 slices) 2 tsp mustard			
potato chips		small bag chips (1 oz)			
skim milk		8 oz skim milk (1 glass)			

Daily food diary

	Blood Glucose Readings			Number of											
	2 hours after	1 hour after	before meals	grams Protein	grams Sat. Fat	grams Total Fat	grams Fiber	milligrams Cholesterol	grams Carbohydrates	Calories	Serving Size	How Cooked	Food Items		
Breakfast/*															
Snack #1/*															
Lunch/*															
Snack #2/*															
Dinner/*															
Snack #3/*															
Daily Totals															

This page may be photocopied by patient. © P&H

* Enter the time you eat each meal or snack.

Dining out

Part of your planning will include meals eaten out. How often you eat out will determine how careful you need to be in your menu choices. The more often you eat out the more closely your choices need to match your meal plan. But, if you eat out very rarely, it may be that you can vary from your plan for just one meal.

If you take insulin, schedule your injections around eating out. Ask your dietitian for ways to adjust your meal plan and insulin injections.

With any change in your meal schedule:

- plan ahead for when you will eat
- know your meal plan and food groups
- know portion sizes for each group
- decide what you are going to order based on your meal plan

Your dietitian can show you how to make your meal plan flexible so you can enjoy dining out, holidays, special occasions, vacations and such.

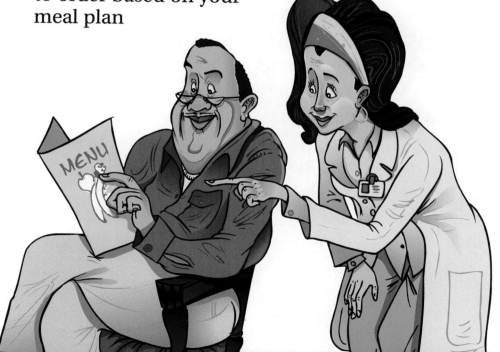

Most of the time, eating out in restaurants means more fat, sugar and calories. So, plan your "meals out" with this in mind. These tips may help:

- Choose broiled, roasted, steamed, poached, blackened, grilled, barbequed or stir fried foods rather than fried, au gratin, creamed, sautéed or buttery ones.
- Choose "heart healthy" or "lite" foods from the menu.
- Ask that salad dressings, mayonnaise, butter, margarine or sour cream be served "on-the-side."
- Order clear soups, like broths or consommé, or vegetable based soups, instead of cream soups.
- Try to avoid salads made with mayonnaise (tuna, bean, chicken, pasta, potato, etc.).
- Choose lettuce salads with raw vegetables or sliced tomatoes.
- Order plain vegetables and ask that no butter or cream sauces be added to them when cooked.
- Order plain bread or rolls, low-fat crackers or melba toast (beware of trans fat in these).
- Don't add salt at the table (ask for a lemon wedge or vinegar to season food, if needed).
- Once you have eaten the amount that makes up a portion, stop (get a "doggy bag" for the rest).
- If portions are large, get a "doggy bag" first, and separate what you will eat from what you take home before you start.

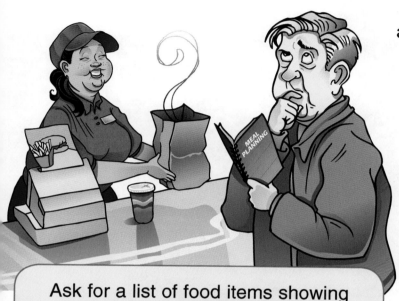

Fast food restaurants are a way of life today. Most fast foods are very high in calories, fat, saturated fat, sodium and sugar. They also tend to not have much fiber. So, when you know you are going to eat fast foods, balance your meal plan that day. Don't let a trip to a fast food restaurant ruin your healthy meal planning.

Ask for a list of food items showing calories, fat, sodium, etc. Also ask what serving sizes are used.

If you mess up, think about taking a brisk walk or go dancing. It takes a lot of exercise to burn off those extra calories, but some exercise will still help lower your blood glucose.

Dining out or entertaining friends and loved ones is something you can enjoy and look forward to. Having diabetes does not have to change this. It may mean, however, that you have to adjust your other meals and snacks that day.

The more you learn about your meal plan and food groups, the easier dining out will be for you. It just takes a little planning.

Doing your part

Your part in healthy meal planning is to make good choices about:

- what you eat
- how much you eat
- when you eat

Here are some tips to help you:

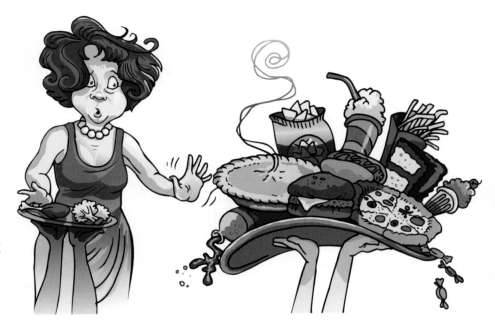

- Keep **track** of the **carbohydrates** you eat (1 serving = 12–15 grams of carbohydrate).

- **Cut down on fatty foods**—bake, broil or grill lean meats and cut away any fat on them.

- **Measure** the foods you eat—know the **serving sizes** (Learn to read food labels, see pages 20–21).

- **Eat every 3–4** hours to help keep your blood glucose level and to help with hunger.

- **Choose** natural foods like **fruits, vegetables** and **whole grains** more often.

- **Limit** eating **canned foods, frozen meals** and most **fast foods** (high in fat, salt and sugar).

- **Eat 5 servings of fruits and vegetables each day.**

Stay Active and Exercise

Another important part of staying healthy is **regular exercise.** Regular means you exercise 3 or more days a week for at least 30 minutes each time.

The best kinds of exercises are those that increase your heart rate. They are called aerobic. Brisk walking, bike riding, swimming or singles tennis are examples. But anything that gets you moving is good for you.

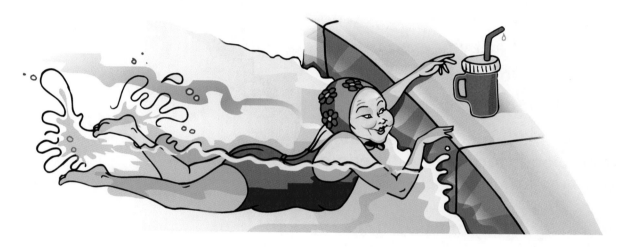

Exercise should be part of your plan because it:

- helps your body use blood glucose faster and better
- helps you manage stress
- gets you in shape
- increases your energy
- helps your diabetes medicine work better
- helps to make you stronger and more flexible
- improves the way you look and feel
- makes it easier to control your weight
- increases your stamina (ability to exercise longer)

Blood glucose and exercise

Your blood glucose reacts to any exercise. How depends on:

- your blood glucose level before you start
- the type of meal you eat before you begin
- the medicine you take and when you take it
- the type of exercise you do
- how hard you exercise
- how long you exercise
- how fit you are

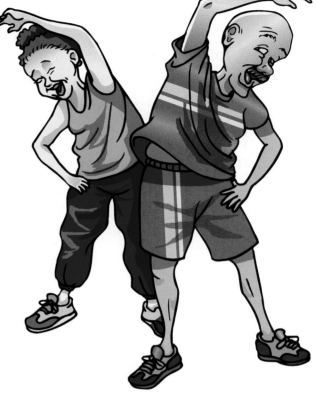

If you take diabetes medicine, your blood glucose can sometimes drop too low during exercise (less than 70 mg/dl). You may get a headache, feel dizzy, shaky or weak. These are signs of hypoglycemia* (low blood glucose).

Warming up before exercise gets your muscles ready to exercise. A good way to warm up is to walk slowly for 5-10 minutes before you begin exercising. Cooling down lets your muscles unwind after you exercise. A good way to cool down is to do the same things you did to warm up.

Always talk with your doctor, nurse or diabetes educator before you begin any exercise program or new activity.

* See pages 55-58 for more about hypoglycemia.

When you exercise, you improve your body's use of insulin, blood glucose and fat. **Learn what effect the exercises you do have on your blood glucose.** And, keep in mind that **exercise can lower your blood glucose for as long as 24 hours afterward.**

Because exercise affects your blood glucose:

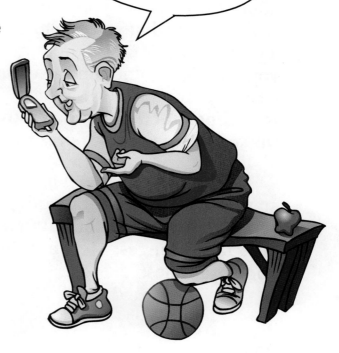

My glucose is o.k. I can keep on exercising!

- **check** it **before** you **exercise** (it should be higher than 100 mg/dl and less than 250 mg/dl)

- **watch for signs** of low blood glucose as you exercise (see page 55)

- **be ready to check** it **during** exercise

- **check** it **after** you exercise

- **carry a snack** (15 g of carbohydrate*) with you in case your blood glucose goes too low

- **carry more than one snack** with you if you are more than 1 hour from home or far from some place to buy a snack

It is best to exercise about 1-3 hours after you eat.

See page 57 for some examples.

The right exercise for you

All exercise is important and there are many types you can do. Yoga, for example, can help reduce stress and help you keep a lean body mass. Weight training increases muscle and causes you to burn more calories during the day.

Talk with your diabetes educator about the activities you like to do. It may be that what you like to do can be a part of your exercise program. If not, you may find something else that is fun, easy and that you might enjoy. The key is to **choose activities you enjoy and make them a regular part of your life.**

The right exercise will help you stay within your target blood glucose range. Ask your doctor or nurse about your target ranges. Here are some good examples:

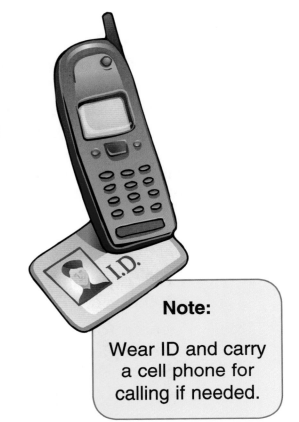

Note:

Wear ID and carry a cell phone for calling if needed.

Fasting (before meals)	70-130 mg/dl
1 to 2 hours after meals	less than 180 mg/dl

Diabetes Medicines

You may have to take some kind of diabetes medicine now or in the future. Whether you have to or not will depend on your body. Diabetes is progressive. That means your body's needs will change as time goes by.

A few people with type 2 diabetes don't need medicine. Others need to take pills, inject insulin or do both. The amount of insulin your pancreas makes may be enough, as long as you stick to your meal plan and exercise. But, over time this may change.

Checking your blood glucose levels on a regular basis will help your doctor or nurse know if you need medicine. It may be that you only need medicine at certain times—like when you're under a lot of stress or when you have an infection.

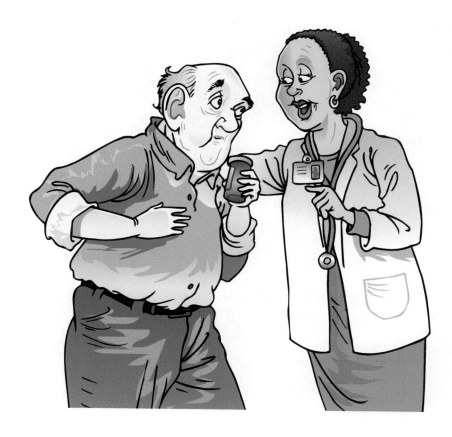

Oral Medicine (pills)

Pills may be needed when diet and exercise alone are not enough to control your diabetes. **But even when you take pills, meal planning and exercise are still very important.**

The right medicine for you is matched to your needs and how your body reacts when you take it. These medicines work best when taken at the same time each day to match the foods you eat.

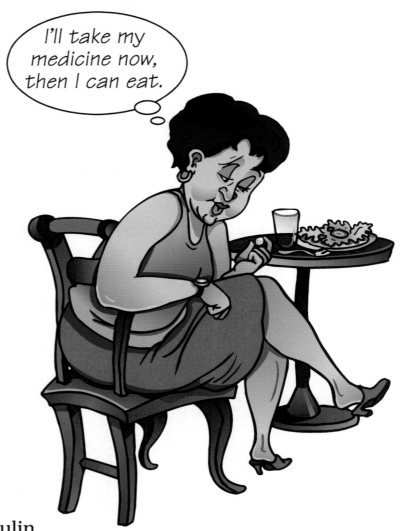

I'll take my medicine now, then I can eat.

All oral diabetes medicines work by reducing blood glucose, but they do it in different ways. None contain insulin. They can be:

- used alone
- in combination with each other
- combined with insulin

The oral medicines that are now available belong to 1 of 6 types. Learn more about them on the next page.

Type of drug	What it does	Generic (Brand Name)
Sulfonylurea (sul-fon-nil-u-ree-a)	helps the pancreas release more insulin and makes it easier for the insulin to work	glyburide (DiaBeta, Micronase) glipizide (Glucotrol or Glucotrol XL) glimepiride (Amaryl)
Meglitinide (me-gli-ti-nide)	helps the pancreas release more insulin	repaglinide (Prandin) nateglinide (Starlix)
Biguanide (bi-gwa-nide)	decreases the liver's release of stored glucose, which makes it easier for insulin to work	metformin (Glucophage, Glucophage XR, Fortamet or Glumetza)
Thiazolidinedione (thi-a-zol-i-deen-di-on)	makes the body's cells more able to use insulin	pioglitazone (Actos TZD's)
Alpha-glucosidase inhibitor (alfa glu-co-side-ace in-hib-it-or)	slows down the digestion of carbohydrates after a meal	acarbose (Precose) miglitol (Glyset)
DPP-4 inhibitor	allows a compound (GLP-1) that reduces blood glucose to remain active longer in the blood	Sitagliptin (Januvia) Saxaglipitin (Onglyza) Linagliptin (Tradjenta)

If your medicine is not listed, it may be new. Ask your doctor how it works. Some of these may put you at risk for low blood glucose. See pages 55–58.

There are also **Combination Therapy Products**	helps the pancreas release more insulin or decreases the liver's release of stored glucose	glyburide and metformin (Glucovance) glipizide and metformin (Metaglip) rosiglitazone and metformin (Avandamet)

Other medicine

Other types of medicines to treat type 2 diabetes are called incretin mimetics and GLP-1 analogs. These are injectable medicines that are most often used along with oral diabetes medicines.

Byetta® (exenatide) is given before your two main meals of the day, at least 6 hours apart. It can be given anytime within 60 minutes (1 hour) of the meal.

Victoza® (liraglutide) is given once every 24 hours.

Both drugs help:

- your pancreas make more insulin

- keep your blood sugar from going too high after you eat

- food move slower through your stomach

- keep your liver from releasing too much glucose into your blood stream after you eat

Pens that are not opened and not being used should be stored in the refrigerator. They are good until the expiration date on the pen. Once opened or used, they may stay at room temperature for about 30 days.

Insulin

Insulin must be injected. It cannot be taken by mouth (it would be digested in your stomach and intestines and never get into your cells). Your doctor, nurse or diabetes educator will teach you when, where, how much and how to inject it.

Injecting insulin gives your body the insulin it either lacks or can't use. But, because insulin removes blood glucose, taking too much can lead to low blood sugar (see pages 55-58).

Here is what you need to know about insulin:

- **the different types**
  - when it starts to work (onset)
  - when it works best (peak action)
  - how long it lasts (duration)
- **the right amount to take** (number of units)
- **ways to inject it** (syringe, pump, pen)
- **how to mix two kinds** (in some cases)
- **where to inject it** (injection sites)
- **how to store it** (refrigerate)
- **when to dispose of it** (30 days after opening)

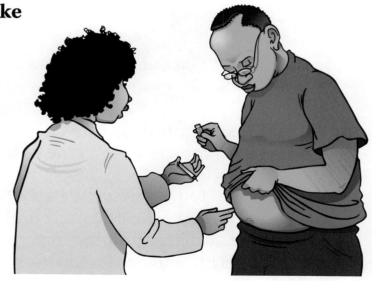

The different types

Insulin is most often **identified by how fast it starts working or how long it works.**

Type	When it starts to work (Onset)	When it's at its best (Peak)	How long it lasts (Duration)	Examples* generic (Brand)
Rapid-acting	15 minutes	30-90 minutes	3-5 hours	(humalog) Lispro or aspart (Novolog) glulisine (Apidra)
Short-acting	½-1 hour	2-4 hours	5-8 hours	regular Humulin R Novolin R
Intermediate-acting	1-3 hours	8 hours	10-16 hours	NPH
Long-acting	5 hours	8-10 hours	Up to 24 hours	Detemir (Levemir)
	1 hour	No peak	24 hours	Glargine (Lantus)

Note: Combinations of these are also available and may be part of your treatment plan.

Insulin is measured in units (labeled "U"). **A unit is always the same, no matter which type of insulin it is.**

In the U.S. today, there are two strengths of insulin used: U-100 and U-500. The one most often used is U-100. But, it may not be available in some foreign countries. So if you travel outside the U.S. and use U-100 insulin, you may need to carry a supply with you. (see travel tips on page 75).

* If your insulin is not listed, it may be new. Ask your doctor how it works.

The right amount to take

Your doctor or nurse will decide:

- how many units of insulin you need and when
- the type and brand to take
- how often to take it
- whether or not you need to mix two kinds of insulin

It may be that you will use one type of insulin every day. But for an emergency, you may use a different type. Or, you may have to take more or less at certain times. All of this is part of your insulin treatment plan.

My insulin treatment plan	
Before breakfast	_____ units of insulin _____ kind of insulin _____ when to take it
Before lunch	_____ units of insulin _____ kind of insulin _____ when to take it
Before dinner	_____ units of insulin _____ kind of insulin _____ when to take it
Before bedtime	_____ units of insulin _____ kind of insulin _____ when to take it

Insulin delivery methods

To use insulin the right way, you need to get it ready and follow the right injection steps. You can use different delivery methods to take insulin:

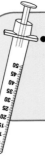

- **disposable insulin syringes** — you draw up the insulin into the syringe and give yourself a shot

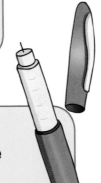

- **pens**— use insulin cartridges in a pen-like device to give the shot

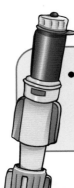

- **needle-free jet injectors**— you inject insulin through the skin by air pressure

- **pumps**— a small device delivers continuous insulin into your body by a thin plastic tube

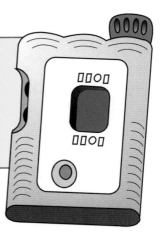

Your doctor, nurse or diabetes educator will explain each type of device, the type of insulin it uses and its cost. Then he or she will work with you to decide which way is best for you. And based on that, will teach you the right way to prepare the insulin and how to inject it.

In some cases you may want to use a pen to inject when you are away from home, but use a syringe when you are at home. The disposable syringe is the least costly method to use. But, using an insulin pen can be useful and convenient.

Disposable syringes

Syringes come in different sizes. And, the length of the needle can vary from 5/16 of an inch to ½ inch. The needle length to use is based on your weight and height. You can also find "fine" and "very fine" needles. The finer the needle, the less you feel the shot.

Insulin pens

There are many different types of insulin pens available. Each one may be a little different in how it is used. A cartridge insulin pen uses an insulin cartridge that allows you to dial up the amount of insulin you need to take. It can be used again. A pre-filled insulin pen contains enough insulin for one injection and then you throw it away. All insulin pens use disposable needles that are used only once and then thrown away. The needles come in varying lengths from 5 millimeters to 12 millimeters. The smallest pen needles are very short and very thin, so you feel the shot less.

Injecting insulin

Get all of your supplies together before you begin. When injecting insulin, **use the same routine each time**. Inject your insulin into the layer of skin just below the outer layer, not into the muscle. Injections in your muscles absorb fast and don't last long.

Insulin is absorbed fastest if injected in your stomach area (abdomen). How fast it is absorbed decreases when injected in your arm, leg and hip areas (in that order). Insulin is used faster during exercise. So, you may want to use your abdomen, rather than an arm or leg, if you are going to exercise soon after injecting.

> If you use your abdomen, inject at least 2 inches away from your belly button and any scars or wounds.

Mixing and injecting 2 kinds of insulin

If you need to inject 2 types of insulin, they are most often mixed and injected at one time. However, some types of insulin are not mixed together. Two syringes or pens must be used in this case.

If you need to take an intermediate acting (NPH) and either a rapid acting (humalog) or short acting (regular) insulin, you can buy some mixed insulins in a pre-filled syringe that you don't have to mix yourself. Your doctor, nurse or diabetes educator will talk with you about the kinds of insulin you need, tell you if you need to mix them and show you how to do it.

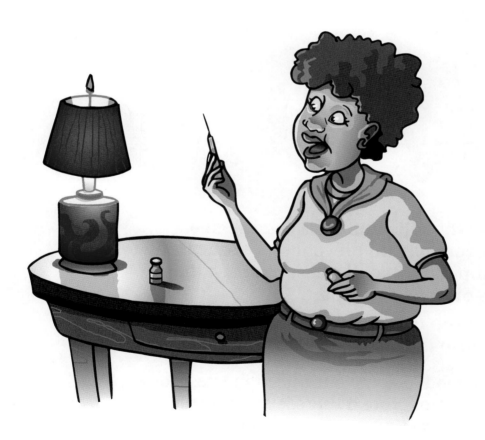

Injection sites

When injecting insulin, follow these rules:

- Choose your injection sites from those shown on the figures. Your doctor, nurse or diabetes educator will help you decide which sites are best for you.

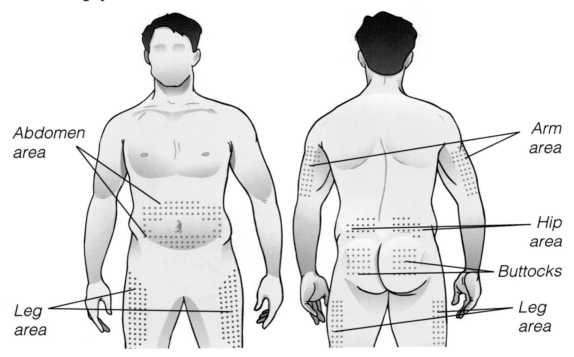

- **Rotate the injection sites** you use in each area **every day** (to prevent scar tissue from developing). A good rule is to space the injections one inch apart.

- Do not rub the injection site after injecting. This can cause the insulin to be absorbed too fast.

- Take a good look at your injection sites from time to time. Note if there is any bruising, redness, infection or thickening of the skin. If so, tell your diabetes educator.

Storing insulin

Always keep one or more extra bottles or pens of insulin on hand at home or on trips. Any form of insulin will fit in a pocket or purse, but never leave insulin where it is very hot (more than 86° F /30°C) or below freezing.

Keep unopened insulin (vials or unused pens) in the refrigerator, but do not freeze. Storing them on the door of the refrigerator will keep them at about 40°F / 4.4°C. Once opened, insulin should be stored at room temperature. (Keep it out of direct sunlight.)

When you open a vial or pen of insulin, write the date on it. Do not use after the expiration date.

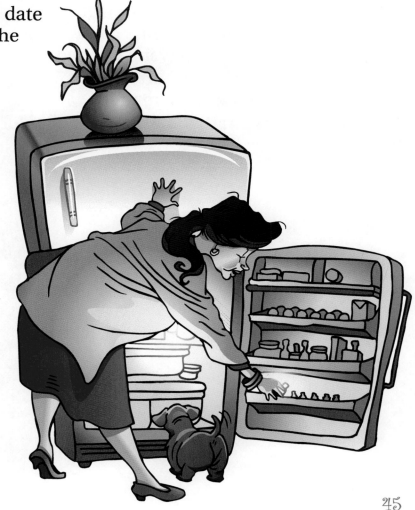

When to dispose of your insulin

Unopened insulin can be stored in the refrigerator door until the expiration date shown on the package. It should not be used beyond the expiration date.

If stored at room temperatures between 60°-85°F (16°-29° C), it can be used for about 1 month. After that, throw away any unused insulin.

Always look at your insulin before you inject it. If it changes color or has any clumps or little specks floating in it, do not use it. These may be signs that the insulin has lost some or all of its strength. If you haven't opened it, you may be able to return it to the pharmacy for exchange (if it's not past the expiration date).

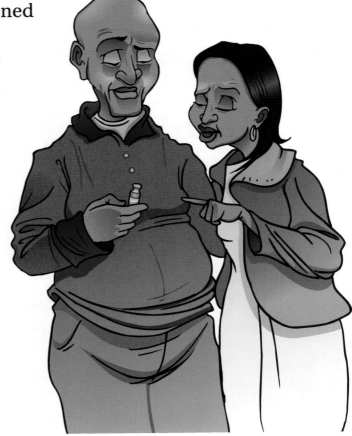

Other diabetes medicine

For those who take insulin, there is another diabetes medicine that can be used along with insulin. It is for adults who have not been able to control blood sugar (glucose) levels with insulin. The type of medicine is called amylin mimetics. People with diabetes do not make enough insulin or amylin. This drug is used with insulin to replace the missing amylin. Using amylin may reduce the amount of insulin you need at meal times. It is not used in place of insulin, but along with it.

Currently there is only one drug of this type in use - Pramlintide acetate (Symlin). It is injected but not in the same syringe that you use to inject insulin. It also comes in a pre-filled pen for injecting. It is injected about 15 minutes before you eat a meal and works to lower blood sugar during the 3 hours after the meal. Your mealtime insulin dose should be reduced by 50 percent when you start Symlin.

Using Symlin helps:

- keep blood sugar from going too high after you eat

- food move more slowly through your stomach

- keep your liver from releasing too much glucose into your blood stream after you eat

- you feel full sooner during meals (helping you eat less, which may lead to weight loss)

Symlin vials and pens that are not opened and not being used should be stored in the refrigerator. They are good until the expiration date on the vial or pen. Once opened, they may stay at room temperature for about 30 days.

Reducing Stress

Reducing stress is an important part of your management plan. **Stress (from emotion or an illness) can cause** your **blood glucose to go up or down.** Most often it will go up.

When you are under stress, your body takes action. Your hormones make a lot of energy for your cells (glucose and fat). However, because you have diabetes, insulin may not be able to get this extra glucose into your cells. It collects in your blood. This makes it harder to keep your blood glucose levels within your target range.

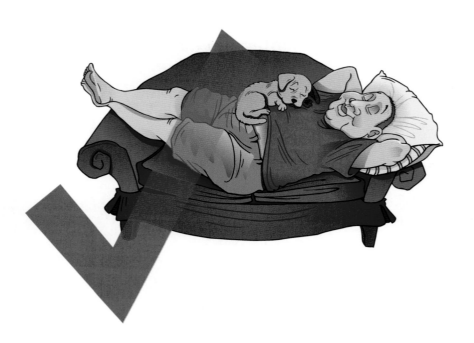

Stress also makes it hard to take good care of yourself. You may not exercise as you should, you may not follow your meal plan or you may forget to test your blood glucose levels. So learning to manage every day stress is a must.

Having diabetes may mean changing some lifestyle habits. And, change causes stress. **Learning to manage the stress** caused by these changes is how you cope. This **involves** either:

- **fixing the problem**
- **getting rid of the problem**
- **learning to live with it**

You have some control over how you react to the stress you face. You can learn to relax, accept what you cannot change or fix problems you have some control over. You can also get help or support from others who have diabetes.

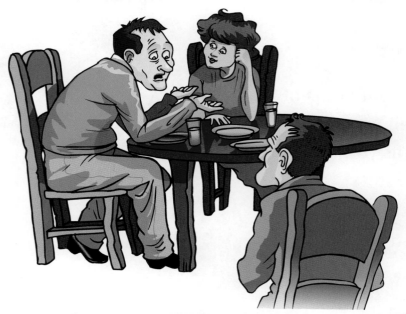

How you choose to manage your stress is up to you. You may not deal with it like someone else would. That's OK. **What's important is that you learn how to manage it in a healthy way.**

Monitoring

Regular self-monitoring is a must when you have diabetes. It is the best way to tell if your diabetes is under control. It includes testing your:

- **blood glucose levels**
- **urine** or **blood** for **ketones**

Testing blood glucose

This test gives information about how your plan is working. Your test results can show if you are:

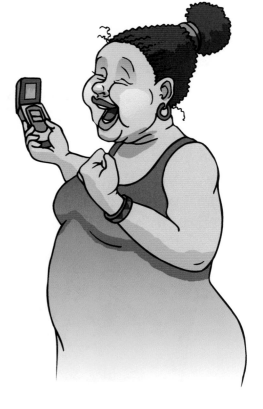

- taking the right amount of medicine
- eating the right amount of food
- eating the right kinds of food
- eating when you should
- exercising as you need to
- managing stress

It's important to monitor your blood glucose and keep it in a normal range.

Fasting (before meals)	70-130 mg/dl
1 to 2 hours after meals	less than 180 mg/dl

How to measure your blood glucose

To measure your blood glucose you need a test kit. Your diabetes educator, doctor or nurse will help you get your first one. It will include:

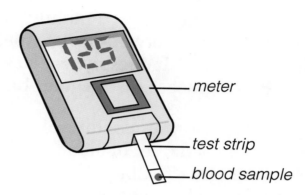

meter

test strip

blood sample

- a test meter
- testing strips
- lancet (to stick your finger to get a drop of blood)
- instructions on how to use the meter
- booklet to record your results

He or she will also teach you how to do self-monitoring. It is important to check at different times of the day. The basic steps involve getting a drop of blood from your finger, arm or leg onto a test strip.* The meter can tell your blood glucose level from that drop of blood.

It is very important that the readings you get each time are right. Your doctor will make changes to your treatment plan based on these. If they are not correct, then your management plan may not be right. You will learn how to check your meter and test strips for quality control.

Some people monitor their blood glucose once a day. Others need to test more often. Ask how often you need to test. **Keep a record of your results and take it to each doctor, nurse or clinic visit.**

* *In the future, this may change. Advances in monitoring methods are being made.*

A1c testing (long-term monitoring)

Another important way to make sure your diabetes management plan is working is with a **Hemoglobin A1c test (A1c)**. This test measures the amount of glucose in your blood over the last 3 months. It is a way for your doctor to have a very up-to-date measure of your blood glucose control. It **does not replace checking your blood glucose on a regular basis**.

For this test, your doctor will draw a small amount of blood from your arm. The blood is then sent to a lab to be tested. The lab will send the results to your doctor.

A good score for this test is 6.5-7 percent or less. Normal is 4-6 percent. A test result of more than 7 percent may mean changes need to be made in your management plan. Learn your score and what it means to you. **A good score can delay or prevent serious problems caused by diabetes.**

Everyone who has type 2 diabetes should have this test **done at least twice a year**. If you take insulin, you should have it done 4 times a year.

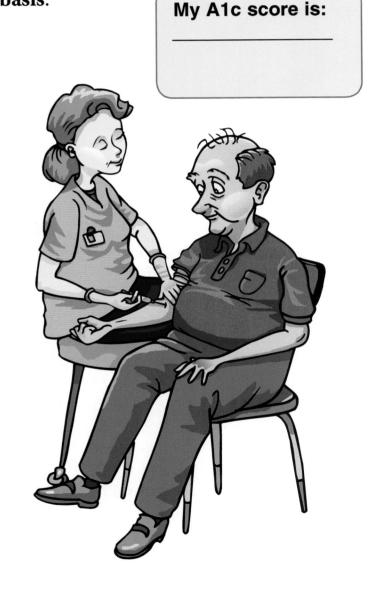

My A1c score is:

_____

Testing for ketones

Another self-monitoring step is to **test for ketones**. There are two ways to do this: urine testing or blood testing. Though done less often than checking blood glucose, it is an important test **if you take insulin or are pregnant.**

Blood ketone testing uses a meter, just like blood sugar testing. The blood test can detect ketones before they get into your urine.

When there is a shortage of insulin, your body breaks down stored fat for energy. As a result, ketones are formed. Large amounts of ketones in your urine or blood means trouble. It can lead to ketoacidosis,* coma or death.

Learn to test for ketones regularly if you are:

- trying to lose weight by reducing calories
- ill or have an infection
- under severe stress
- involved in a trauma (like a car wreck)
- pregnant

*If you have signs of **ketoacidosis** (a dangerous condition), check your blood glucose level.

These are the signs to look for:

- shortness of breath
- nausea or vomiting
- dry mouth
- fruity smelling breath
- stiff muscles
- frequent urination
- dry or flushed skin

Call your nurse or doctor right away and drink fluids without sugar or caffeine. Avoid getting dehydrated.

Otherwise, test your urine or your blood if you show signs of having **high blood glucose (300 mg/dl or higher).** And, don't get upset if one urine test shows ketones. Test again 4 hours later. Your doctor, nurse or diabetes educator will tell you about ketone testing, what materials are needed and how to get them.

Diabetes complications

Even when you are managing your diabetes, sometimes problems can occur. Some are short term (or acute) and others are long term (or chronic). Some of these will not disable you nor last forever. They may appear at any time and can be fixed.

However, some complications can be crippling and may not be fixable. Know about all that can happen. And, learn how to avoid as many as you can.

Short-Term Problems

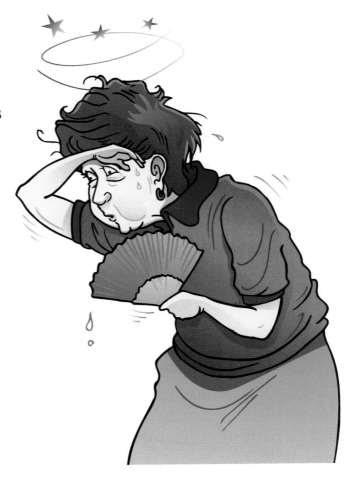

Short term signals may be a warning sign. They may tell you to tighten your blood glucose control before it ends up being more serious.

The two most common acute problems are:

- **hypoglycemia**
  (low blood glucose)
- **hyperglycemia**
  (high blood glucose)

Hypoglycemia (low blood glucose)

Sometimes, the level of glucose in your blood goes too low **(below 70 mg/dl)**. This is called hypoglycemia or low blood glucose. With low blood glucose, you don't have enough energy. It can be very dangerous and can even lead to coma.

You may have low blood glucose from time to time. The best thing to do is take fast action when you feel it coming on. Know your signs and what lowers your blood glucose. Remember that exercise, insulin and oral medicines lower blood glucose, and food raises it.

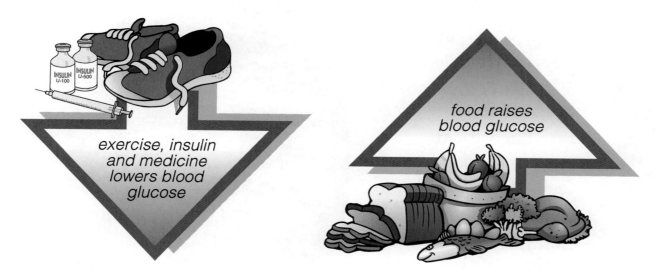

food raises blood glucose

exercise, insulin and medicine lowers blood glucose

To prevent low blood glucose, stay on top of managing your diabetes:

- Take the amount of insulin or oral medicine prescribed.
- Don't miss a meal or eat off schedule.
- Don't exercise without planning ahead.
- Don't drink too much alcohol.
- Try to stay healthy, but if you get sick, follow your sick day plan (see pages 61-62).
- Balance the food you eat with the medicine you take.

Tell family members, close friends, teachers and people at work that you have diabetes. Tell them the signs and symptoms so they will know when your blood glucose is low. Show them what to do, if you can't treat yourself. Here is what to look for:

- dizziness or headache
- being very hungry
- mood changes
- feeling weak all over or having trouble using your muscles
- being confused or not thinking clearly
- feeling nervous, shaky or irritable
- rapid heartbeat
- cold, clammy feeling or pale skin
- sweating too much
- numbness, tingling in the mouth or on the tongue
- passing out (in severe cases)

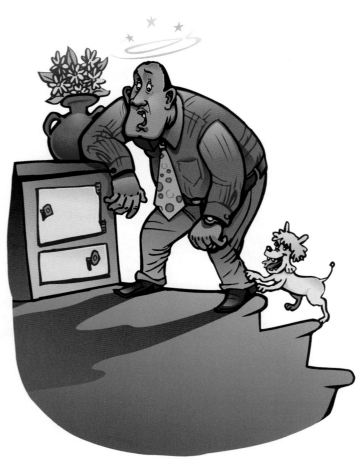

The level at which you feel your blood glucose is low may be different than it is for someone else.

When you feel that your glucose is low, check it. If it is below 70 mg/dl, **take 15 grams of quick-acting carbohydrate** right away. Choose 1 of these:

- drink **4-6 oz of regular** (non-diet) **soda** or **8 oz of skim milk**
- drink **½ cup (or 4 oz) of fruit juice** (orange, apple, grape, etc.)
- take **3-4 glucose tablets** (get these at your pharmacy)
- eat **5-7 pieces of hard candy like Lifesavers®** (not chocolate)

Then rest for 15 minutes and recheck your blood glucose again. If it is still low (less than 70 mg/dl) or if you are still having symptoms, eat or drink another 15 grams of carbohydrates.

If you don't have a meal or snack planned for 1 hour or more, eat a light snack with 30 g of carbs or 15 g of carbs with some protein.

If your blood glucose is lower than it was to start with, call your doctor or nurse.

If you can't swallow a fast acting carb, someone will need to give you a shot of glucagon and call for help. **Glucagon** is a prescription medicine that **raises blood glucose.** It is injected just like insulin. If you take insulin, you should have a glucagon kit handy. Teach those around you when and how to use it, too.

Don't wait to treat low blood glucose. It is not safe! You may pass out. If you get confused, pass out or have a seizure, you need help fast. Don't try to drive yourself if this happens. Someone else may need to take you to the hospital.

A good reason to share the information in this book with your family is so they know your signs of low blood sugar and can help quickly.

Because low blood glucose may happen from time to time, always carry ID when you are away from home to tell others you have diabetes (see page 76).

Hyperglycemia (high blood glucose)

When glucose does not go into your cells, it builds up in your blood. This leads to **hyperglycemia or high blood glucose (over 200 mg/dl).**

As blood glucose levels increase, your body loses a lot of fluid. You can become dehydrated.

To prevent high blood glucose:

- don't eat more than you should
- eat at the same time each day
- control stress
- exercise regularly
- take insulin and/or oral medicine when you should and in the amount you should
- don't take other medicines that can affect your blood glucose
- stay on top of managing your diabetes
- try to stay healthy, but if you get sick, follow your sick day plan (see page 61-62).

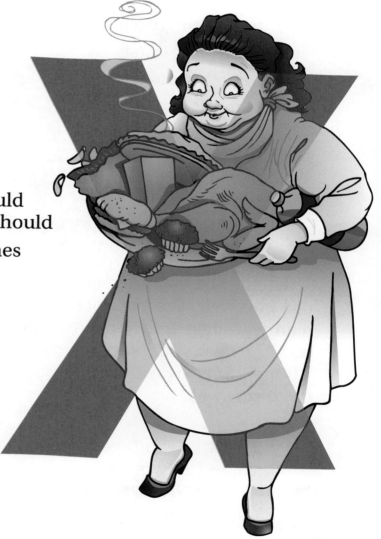

Knowing you have high blood glucose is very important. You want to **avoid it when you can but be prepared when it happens.** When you first begin to have signs, do something about it to help avoid serious problems.

Here are the signs to watch for:

- being hungry a lot
- being very thirsty
- urinating often
- being very tired or sleepy
- having stomach pains or nausea
- losing weight without trying to
- hard to heal wounds or having infections often

Even when you are managing your diabetes well, it can happen. Drink plenty of sugar-free fluids (8 oz every hour). Check your blood glucose every 4 hours. Stay away from sick people and try to stay well.

Diabetes is progressive and your needs can change. **Call your primary caregiver when your blood glucose is over 200 mg/dl three times in a row.** You may need a change in your treatment plan.

When You Are Sick

Being sick can make it hard for you to keep your blood glucose levels within your target range. They may go up. Vomiting and diarrhea, along with high blood sugar can cause you to lose too much fluid. You may easily become dehydrated. Being sick may also make it hard to:

- stick with your meal plan
- exercise
- take your medicine as you should

While you are sick, continue your treatment plan as best you can. You want to avoid any further problems.

Call your doctor or nurse if you have:

- been sick or had a fever (more than 101.5°F/38.3°C) for a few days and are not getting better
- diarrhea or vomiting that lasts longer than 6 hours
- moderate to large amounts of ketones in your urine
- blood glucose levels higher than 200 mg/dl or less than 70 mg/dl
- symptoms of ketoacidosis (see page 53)
- symptoms you can't explain

Over-the-counter cold and cough medicines may affect your blood glucose. Check with your doctor or pharmacist about safe ones. Keep some on hand in case of illness.

A Sick Day Plan

Use this sick day plan to help keep your blood glucose levels as close to normal as you can.

- **rest**
- **drink** a lot of **fluids** (8 oz every hour) unless you are told not to
  - if your blood glucose is over 240 mg/dl, use sugar-free drinks like broth, tea or water
  - if your blood glucose is less than 240 mg/dl, drink fluids that have 10 - 15 grams of carbohydrates in them
- try your best to **stick with your normal meal plan** (but, if you can't, try to eat 45 - 50 grams of carbohydrates every 3 - 4 hours)
- **if you can't eat** at all, **try a** carbohydrate **liquid** or near liquid, like:
  - ½ cup regular soda
  - ½ cup sherbet
  - 1 Popsicle®
  - ½ cup gelatin
- **test** your **blood glucose every 3 - 4 hours** (test your urine for ketones, too)
- **take your medicine** (insulin and/or pills) even if you can't eat (If you are not eating, ask your nurse if you need to take less medicine.)
- call your doctor if you have 3 blood glucose readings in a row over 200 mg/dl

Some food and fluids that have 10-15 carbohydrate grams:

- 1 cup Gatorade
- 1 cup milk
- ½ cup ginger ale or soft drink
- 1 cup tomato juice
- 6 vanilla wafers
- 1 slice of toast/ bread
- ½ cup cooked cereal
- ½ cup ice cream
- 6 saltine crackers
- 1 cup chicken noodle soup
- ½ cup cottage cheese with fruit
- ½ cup juice

Long-Term (Chronic) Problems

Chronic problems tend to happen over a period of years. If blood glucose is not controlled your risk is even greater. Chronic problems include:

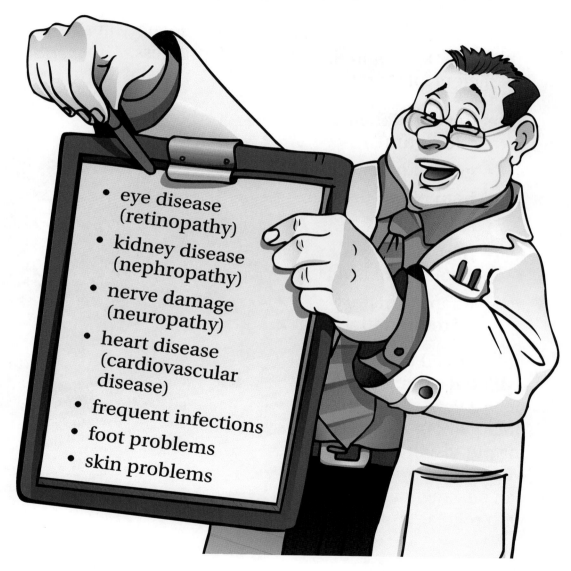

- eye disease (retinopathy)
- kidney disease (nephropathy)
- nerve damage (neuropathy)
- heart disease (cardiovascular disease)
- frequent infections
- foot problems
- skin problems

Your risk of developing these problems can be reduced. **The better you manage** your diabetes, **the less risk you have.**

Eye disease (Retinopathy)

Diabetes is the leading cause of blindness in the U.S. for adults over age 20. The most common eye problem for people with type 2 diabetes is **diabetic retinopathy** (damage or disease of the retina).

The less you manage your diabetes the more at risk you are for this. And the more it will progress. Other risk factors for it are:

- having diabetes a long time
- getting older
- high blood pressure
- smoking
- high blood cholesterol levels
- a family history of retinopathy

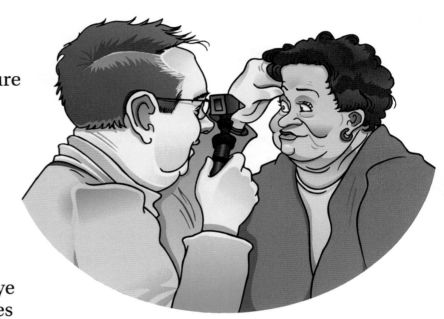

You need to **have a dilated retinal exam once a year**. Tell your eye doctor about any changes in your vision at each visit. Many other eye problems can be caught and prevented with regular visits.

Kidney disease (Nephropathy)

Your kidneys filter the waste products from your blood and pass them out through your urine. This is a very important job.

Diabetes is the most common cause of kidney disease. It is found by checking for **microalbumin** (small amount of protein) in the urine. As a rule, in healthy kidneys, no protein is found in the urine.

Kidney disease is linked to poor diabetes management—namely high blood glucose. As blood glucose levels increase, it can damage the kidneys. Then more waste products build up in the blood and are not passed out in urine. This can lead to kidney failure. Your risk for getting it also increases the longer you have diabetes. Other risk factors for this disease are:

- frequent urinary tract infections
- uncontrolled high blood pressure
- high blood cholesterol
- smoking

You may have kidney disease and not know it because your kidneys work fine until it is almost too late. Because you have diabetes, be good to your kidneys. **Have a urine test at least once a year to check for microalbumin**.

At the first sign of a urinary tract infection, call your doctor or nurse.

Nerve damage (Neuropathy)

Your risk for nerve damage is greater because you have diabetes. The longer you have diabetes, the greater the risk.

The small blood vessels that feed your nerves can become blocked and cause poor circulation. It may occur after years of poor blood glucose control.

The symptoms can affect any nerve in your body. (Although, more often the feet and lower legs are affected.) It can also affect your bowel, bladder and sexual function. The most common symptoms are:

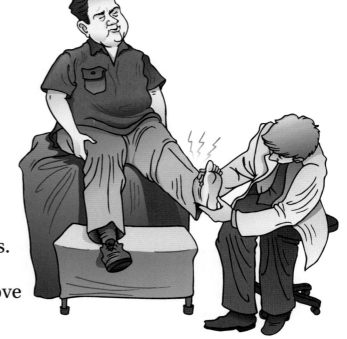

- pain
- numbness (loss of feeling)
- tingling sensation (pins and needles)
- feeling like your legs or feet are "on fire" or "hot"

Tell your doctor or nurse if you have any symptoms. All forms of neuropathy can give you problems. But, most of the time they are not permanent. Symptoms can improve or disappear. Don't ignore them.

Take your shoes and socks off at each visit so your doctor or nurse can examine your feet and legs. They may use a soft wire device (called a monofilament) to test the feeling in your feet and legs.

Heart disease (Cardiovascular Disease)

Heart disease happens when not enough blood and oxygen get through to your heart. It is caused by too much cholesterol and plaque (fatty deposits) building up in your blood vessels and blocking blood flow.

You are 2 to 4 times more likely to develop cardiovascular disease (like heart attack or stroke) than someone who does not have diabetes. This is due, in part, to:

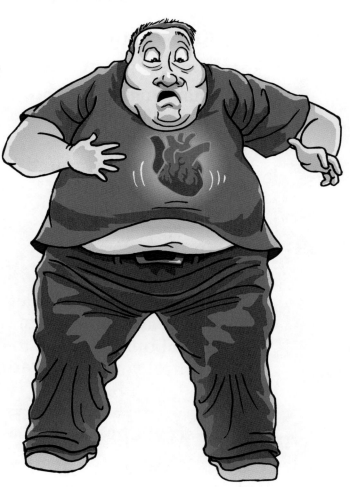

- insulin resistance
- high blood pressure
- obesity
- higher cholesterol and fat levels in your blood

Because diabetes increases the levels of cholesterol and fat in your blood, **more than 75% of people with uncontrolled diabetes die from some form of heart disease.**

To help reduce your risks:

- keep your blood glucose level within your target range
- control what you eat, how much you eat and when you eat
- exercise regularly
- keep your weight in a healthy range
- if you have high blood pressure, (140/80 and higher) keep it under control
- don't smoke or be around others who are smoking because nicotine narrows blocked vessels
- if your cholesterol levels are high, reduce the fat and cholesterol in your diet (if needed, ask your doctor or nurse about medicine to help control your cholesterol)

Target Cholesterol Levels	
Total Cholesterol	less than 200
HDL (Good Cholesterol)	
men	over 40
women	over 50
LDL (Bad Cholesterol)	less than 100
Triglycerides	less than 150

Frequent infections

White blood cells fight infection. When you have uncontrolled diabetes your white blood cells don't work as well. Because of this, you are more likely to get an infection. Poor diabetes control may be the cause. But good blood glucose control can help your white blood cells work better.

Learn the signs of an infection and notify your doctor or nurse if you have any of them:

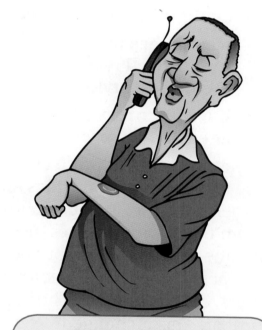

- a sore or wound that is tender to the touch
- pus or mucus draining from a sore or wound
- redness or discoloration of the area around a sore
- skin around area that is warm to the touch
- hardening of skin
- running a fever over 101°F (38.3°C)

Any infection is cause for concern. If your blood glucose levels are not controlled, you will not heal as fast as usual. So it is important that you keep your blood glucose levels within your target range.

Prevention Tip:
Get an annual flu shot and ask your doctor or nurse if you should have a pneumonia vaccine.

Foot problems

When you have diabetes, small problems with your feet can quickly become big problems if not treated the right way. They can even lead to amputation (having your foot or leg taken off).

To take good care of your feet:

- **check your feet each day**
- **avoid injury to your feet**
- **wear shoes (and socks) that fit well** (even if not the newest style)
- **have your feet examined** at each doctor visit

When you check your feet, look at the top, bottom, both sides and in between each toe. If you can't see the bottom of your foot or toes, use a mirror or ask someone to check them for you. Check for any red, cracked or dry areas, sores, ingrown toenails, blisters, cuts or fungus. Check the feeling in your feet. Has it changed? Nerve damage and narrowed blood vessels can cause foot problems.

Call your doctor if you have any redness, blisters, sores or scratches. These injuries can get worse quickly if not treated the right way.

Follow these rules for good foot care:

- File your nails right after you wash and dry your feet. Don't cut into the corners. Do not use toenail clippers, scissors or a knife. Shorten your nails only with an emery board or nail file.

- If you have poor eyesight or trouble reaching your feet, have someone else trim your nails (like a foot doctor).

- Don't cut corns or calluses. Don't use corn plasters or liquid corn or callus removers. Ask your doctor how to use a pumice stone to gently rub them.

- Don't use antiseptic solutions, other remedies and treatments or tape on your feet.

- Wash your feet each day. Use a mild soap and warm (not hot) water. Test your bath water with your hand to make sure it is not too hot. Pat your feet dry. Be sure to dry between your toes well.

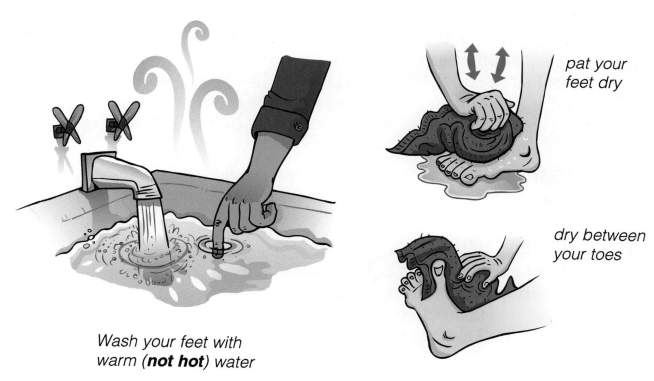

pat your feet dry

dry between your toes

*Wash your feet with warm (**not hot**) water*

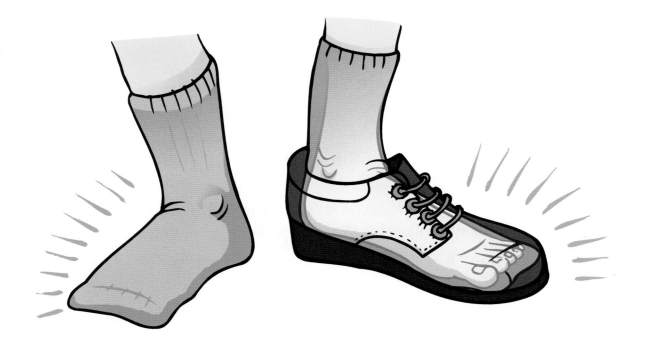

- Ask your doctor to do a "socks off" check of your feet at every visit (at least 2 times a year).

- Always wear shoes and socks. Don't ever go barefoot—not even indoors, at the beach or around the swimming pool.

- Wear shoes that fit well with cushioned insoles and soles. Leather and canvas are best. Do not wear sandals or shoes with open toes or heels. Make sure there are no torn linings, rough areas or objects that don't belong in your shoe (feel inside before you put them on to be sure).

- Wear clean stockings or cotton socks. During cold weather, wear fleece-lined shoes. Wear extra socks if your feet are cold. Wear socks at night to keep your feet warm.

- Don't use hot water bottles, heating pads, battery-powered foot warmers or electric blankets. Protect your feet from extreme heat and cold. Don't get too much sun on your feet.

Skin problems

High blood glucose may lead to dehydration (lack of fluid) or poor blood flow in your feet and legs. This can lead to drying and cracking of the skin.

High blood glucose levels and poor circulation also increase your risk for infection. And, infections increase your blood glucose level and the need for insulin. So avoiding infections and keeping your blood glucose within your target range is important for both preventing and treating skin problems.

Tell your doctor if you have any sign of a skin ulcer (wound) that lasts for more than one day. **If you cut or scrape your skin**, clean the area right away. If it does not begin to heal in 48 hours, ask your doctor or nurse what you need to do. Because you may be more likely to get an infection, these should be **treated right away.**

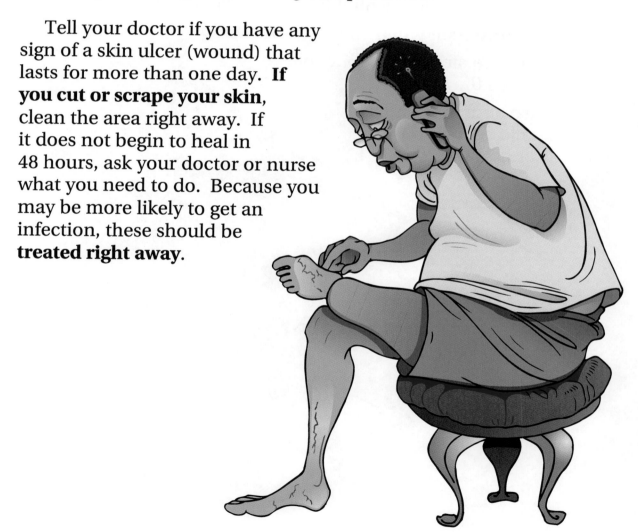

To take good care of your skin:

- eat a well balanced, healthy diet—follow your meal plan

- drink plenty of fluids

- avoid injury to your skin

- keep your skin clean and dry

- pat your skin dry instead of rubbing it

- use a moisturizing lotion (not oil based) that does not contain alcohol (lanolin is good)

- use sunscreen when you go in the sun

- don't use alcohol on your skin (it dries the skin)

- wash your skin with a mild soap and warm (not hot) water

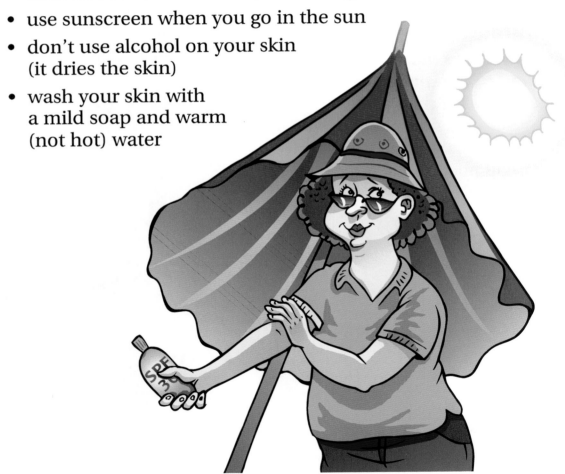

Other things you need to know

Traveling

Always **plan ahead for travel.** Will travel plans interfere with your need to eat at the same time each day? If so, take food and snacks with you. If you take insulin, it should not get too hot or too cold. Do your travel plans affect this? How often do you need to check your blood glucose? Will traveling affect this? Will time zone changes affect the timing of your medicines and meals?

Ask your doctor, nurse or diabetes educator about setting up a travel plan. Your travel plan should also include what to do if you get sick or injured while traveling.

Carry your diabetes supplies with you. Have **extra medicine and supplies** in case you break something. Don't check them in your baggage. If your baggage is lost, you may not be able to replace them quickly. Or, you may not know where to go to get more. Carry a quick-acting carb snack for treating low blood glucose with you too. Make up a "travel kit." Have a checklist for what to include in it.

Note:
Federal aviation guidelines require a person with diabetes to follow certain instructions for passing through checkpoints and screenings. To find out what these are, visit www.tsa.gov. Then click on "Traveler Information," followed by "Disabilities and Medical Conditions." Scroll down and click on "Have Diabetes."

Medical ID

In case of an emergency, **always carry some form of ID*** to let others know you have diabetes. There are bracelets, anklets or necklaces that you wear. Or, you can carry a card in your wallet.

Check with your doctor, nurse, diabetes educator or pharmacy about getting an ID. Another source may be a jewelry store. Or, you can order ID's on the internet

Medic Alert is one type of ID you can buy. It comes as a bracelet or a necklace and has your medical condition and a code number on it. Your medical records are stored under this code number. For more information, call 1-800-432-5378 or visit www.medicalert.org.

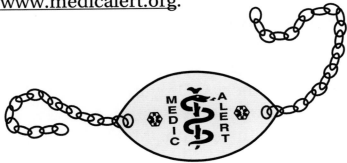

Other sources for medical ID include:

- **Life Alert**
  1-800-360-0329
- **Life Tag**
  1-888-LIFETAG
  www.lifetag.com

Pregnancy

If you are a woman, your diabetes needs to be in very good control before you become pregnant. Your unborn child can be harmed if your diabetes is not controlled. And your pregnancy may not be as healthy. If you are planning on having a baby, **talk with your doctor or nurse before you get pregnant.**

Pregnancy can create complications for any woman. With diabetes it may change the need for insulin and the amount of it you need, as well as your meal plan. You may need to stop taking oral pills and temporarily switch to insulin. You will work closely with your doctor if you become pregnant.

If you do not want to get pregnant talk with your doctor or nurse about birth control.

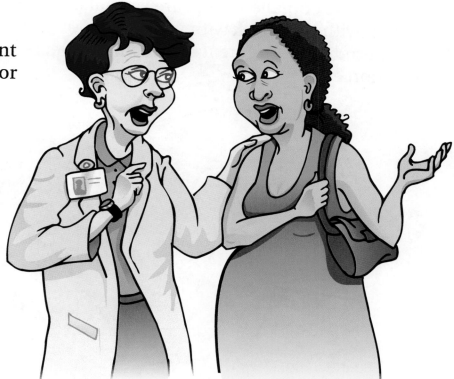

Sexual Concerns

Over time, high blood glucose can lead to nerve damage and poor circulation. This can affect your sex life.

For men...

It can lead to impotence (trouble getting an erection). In some cases, impotence may be a side effect of a medicine you are taking. Or it could be hormonal. There are things that can be done about impotence. Talk with your doctor or nurse about this problem if it happens.

For women...

It can cause less vaginal fluid and frequent infections. Vaginal dryness can be caused by less blood flow to a woman's sex organs. There are special lubricants or gels to help with this. Talk with your doctor or nurse about these products. And treat any vaginal or yeast infection early.

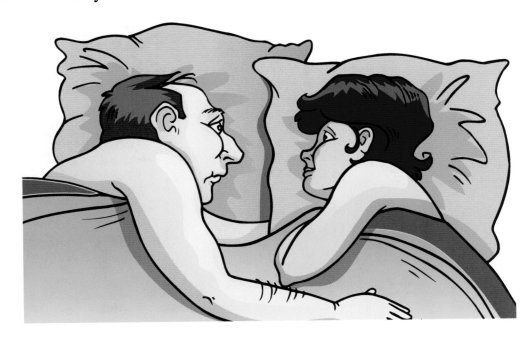

Weight Control

If you are overweight (BMI* between 25 and 29) and have type 2 diabetes, the extra fat makes it harder for your body's insulin to work. Having **extra fat makes it more likely that you will need insulin or pills to control** your **blood glucose**. It also puts you at greater risk for some of the complications of diabetes, like heart disease or stroke. Losing just 10-15 pounds can improve your body's use of its insulin.

Control your weight by following your meal plan and exercising. As you start to balance what you eat with how active you are, you will have a weight change. You'll lose weight if you eat less than your body needs for activities. You'll gain weight if you eat more.

Ask your doctor, nurse or dietitian to help you set a good weight goal. You are more likely to keep weight off if you lose it slowly (1 or 2 pounds a week). If you have trouble losing weight, there are resources that can help. Ask your doctor, dietitian or diabetes educator about these.

> You should not take diet pills or try a "fad" diet to lose weight. These don't work and can affect your diabetes control.

* See page 80 for a BMI (body mass index) Chart.

Your body mass index* (BMI) is a way to tell if you are overweight. It uses your height and weight to give you an index number. The index describes your weight condition.

> 21-24 ....normal healthy weight
> 25-29 ....overweight
> 30 or higher .....obese

To use this chart, follow these steps:

1. Find your height in the first column.

2. Look across that line and find your weight (if you are between 2 numbers, use the closest).

3. Read BMI score at the top of the column.

Your Height	Your BMI score is: 21	22	23	24	25	26	27	28	29	30	31
	Your Weight (pounds)										
4'11"	104	109	114	119	124	128	133	138	143	148	153
5'	107	112	118	123	128	133	138	143	148	153	158
5'1"	111	116	122	127	132	137	143	148	153	158	164
5'2"	115	120	126	131	136	142	147	153	158	164	169
5'3"	118	124	130	135	141	146	152	158	163	169	175
5'4"	122	128	134	140	145	151	157	163	169	174	180
5'5"	126	132	138	144	150	156	162	168	174	180	186
5'6"	130	136	142	148	155	161	167	173	179	186	192
5'7"	134	140	146	153	159	166	172	178	185	191	198
5'8"	138	144	151	158	164	171	177	184	190	197	203
5'9"	142	149	155	162	169	176	182	189	196	203	209
5'10"	146	153	160	167	174	181	188	195	202	209	216
5'11"	150	157	165	172	179	186	193	200	208	215	222
6'	154	162	169	177	184	191	199	206	213	221	228
6'1"	159	166	174	182	189	197	204	212	219	227	235
6'2"	163	171	179	186	194	202	210	218	225	233	241
6'3"	168	176	184	192	200	208	216	224	232	240	248
6'4"	172	180	189	197	205	213	221	230	238	246	254

* from the National Heart, Lung and Blood Institute

Smoking

Smoking is not healthy for anyone, not just those with diabetes. But for you, the risk of heart disease, eye problems and neuropathy are even greater if you smoke. And it also increases your risk of getting cancer and emphysema (a lung disease).

Smoking makes your blood vessels constrict (get tighter) and reduces blood flow. The longer you have diabetes the more likely you are to have reduced blood flow anyway. So smoking compounds your problems.

Quitting may be hard. If so, get help. Ask your doctor or nurse about nicotine replacement therapy (NRT) aids. There are patches, gums, inhalers, nasal sprays, lozenges and pills to help you quit. Stop smoking clinics may also be available in your community.

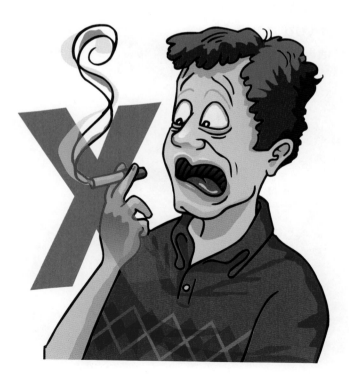

Dental Care

This is good dental care for everyone:

- See your dentist every 6 months for routine cleaning and exams.
- Brush after each meal and floss your teeth each day.

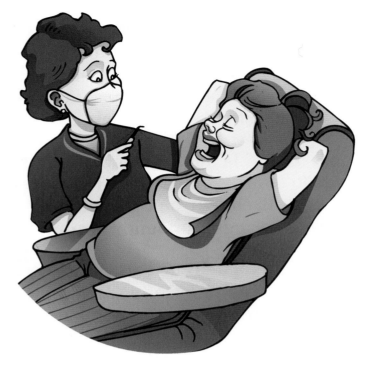

Tell your dentist you have diabetes. You may be more prone to having gum disease. And, gum disease can cause you to lose your teeth.

So, ask your dentist if there is anything special you need to do. Then write that in this chart.

My special dental needs:

Alcohol Use*

The same rules that apply to those who don't have diabetes, apply to you. (This is only if your blood glucose levels are kept within your target range.) Men should have no more than 2 drinks per day. Women should have no more than 1 per day. **Always eat something when you drink alcohol.**

Alcohol does not require insulin for it to be used as an energy source. It is not changed into glucose. Because it can not be used as a source of glucose, **low blood glucose can happen when you drink alcohol without eating food with it.** (It can mask your usual symptoms of low blood glucose.)

One alcoholic drink equals 2 fat servings. It should be substituted for fat servings or fat calories in your meal plan. And, many mixed drinks are made with fruit juice, soft drinks, cream or other products. These need to be counted in your meal plan, too. Extra amounts of alcohol become fat. So if you are trying to lose weight, be aware that alcohol contains calories.

One drink is:

- 1½ oz of liquor
- 5 oz of wine
- 12 oz of beer (lite or regular)

Alcohol and some medicines don't mix. Ask your pharmacist about drinking alcohol if you take any medicine.

* Ask your doctor, nurse, diabetes educator or dietitian if you can have alcohol in your meal plan.

Depression

It may seem that there is a lot for you to know and do when you have diabetes. Having a chronic condition is not easy. At times, it can seem overwhelming. You may feel like giving up and not taking care of yourself. You may become angry or even deny that you have diabetes.

Many people who have diabetes have these feelings at one time or another. It is called depression. And, it can affect your life and your health. Here are some other signs that might mean you are depressed:

- losing weight without trying to
- feeling sad or empty most of the time
- being tired all the time or having no energy (and not having high blood glucose levels)
- feeling worthless, on edge or being irritable a lot
- thinking about death or dying a lot or wanting to end your life
- gaining weight
- trouble sleeping
- sleeping too much
- not wanting to do anything, go anywhere or not enjoying things you used to
- trouble thinking straight, unable to make a decision

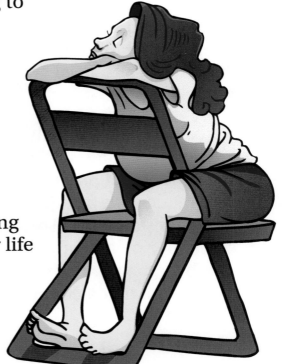

Talk with your doctor, nurse or diabetes educator about any of these feelings you are having. The good news is there are ways to treat depression. There are also medicines (antidepressants) that may help.

The first step is to admit that you are depressed. Then do something about it.

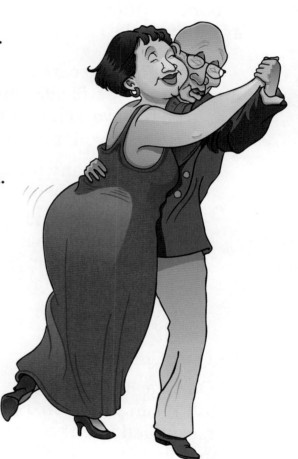

- Get it out and talk about it. This way it doesn't seem so bad.

- Think about all the positives in your life.

- Make time for rest and relaxation. Relax for at least a half hour before you go to bed and get plenty of sleep.

- Find something you like to do and do it. Take a hot bath, get a massage, have a mud bath, go fishing or dancing, sit in a sauna, read a good book.

- Do some physical activity. When you exercise, your body makes natural antidepressants (endorphins). This helps you relax and feel good.

- Make time for fun. Having a few hours of fun to look forward to each week can make a big difference in the way you feel and your attitude.

- Stick to your healthy meal plan. When you eat right you feel better and are better able to deal with depression.

Follow-up care

Once you are on a schedule, your doctor or nurse will want to see how your treatment plan is working. At first you may have follow-up visits often. Then while you are adjusting to your meal plan and medicine, follow-up visits may be every 3 months. After that, you will most likely have checkups every 6 months.

Your **follow-up care is based on your needs**. Your doctor or nurse will talk with you about how often you need to have a checkup. It is very important for you to keep your follow-up visits to see:

- if you have any problems with your glucose level being too high or too low

- if you need to change your meal plan or the amount of medicine (if any) you take each day

- how best to help you adjust to having diabetes

On page 88 is a diabetes diary. It can show you, your doctor, nurse or dietitian if your treatment plan is working. Make a copy and fill it in for 2 weeks. Take it with you to your next follow up visit. Go over it in detail with your doctor, nurse or dietitian.

Your part in managing diabetes

The part you play is to do the best job you can in following your meal plan, exercising on a regular basis, taking your medicine, monitoring your blood glucose and managing the stress in your life. **You are the central player on your diabetes team.** Your doctor, nurse, diabetes educator or dietitian can help set up your plan, but you control it day to day.

Both the quality of your life as well as the length of your life are important. And there is only one reason to learn everything you can about diabetes—to keep you as healthy as possible.

Diabetes is complex. There must be a balance in your treatment. Too much food may increase your blood glucose and mean you need more insulin. Less food or more exercise may reduce your blood glucose. Being stressed can raise or lower your blood glucose.

There is no cure for diabetes yet. So continue to learn all you can about it through reading, local support groups and programs. New research yields new knowledge and treatment options all the time. **Take control of your treatment plan and** work with your diabetes team to **manage your diabetes** and improve your health. You can learn **to live well** with diabetes. **You** can **make the difference**. It really is up to you.

Diabetes diary

My healthy blood glucose range is

before meals: _____ to _____

2 hrs after meals: _____ to _____

at bedtime: _____ to _____

name _____

Date	Meal Plan*							Medicines*			Blood Glucose*				Notes
	Breakfast	Snack 1	Lunch	Snack 2	Dinner	Snack 3	*Exercise	(dose ___)	(dose ___)	(dose ___)	Breakfast	Lunch	Dinner	Bedtime	

*Meal Plan

Followed meal plan	= 0
Varied plan a little	= 1
Varied plan a lot	= 2

*Exercise

No exercise	= 0
Light exercise (20 min or less)	= 1
Moderate exercise (20-45 min)	= 2
Heavy exercise (45+ min)	= 3

*Medicines

Write in exact dosage taken and the time

*Blood Glucose

Write in blood glucose level before meal and 2 hours after

Notes / Questions

Include signs of problems, medication reactions, how meals or activities varied from planned, etc.

Questions and notes

If you have any questions to ask your doctor or nurse, write them down so you don't forget them. Use this space for that. Here's an example:

Q I've always cut my own toenails. Why do I need a doctor to do that?

A

Q

A

Q

A

Resources

American Association of Diabetes Educators
(800) 338-3633
diabeteseducator.org

American Diabetes Association (ADA)
(800) 342-2383
diabetes.org

American Dietetic Association
(800) 877-1600
eatright.org

Cooking Healthy Across America
Order from American Dietetic Association (see above)

Order this book from:

PRITCHETT & HULL ASSOCIATES, INC.
3440 OAKCLIFF RD NE STE 110
ATLANTA GA 30340-3006

Write for our catalog of other
product descriptions and prices.

2014 Edition

Published and distributed by:
Pritchett & Hull Associates, Inc.

Printed in the U.S.A.

This book is only to help you learn.
It is not a substitute for advice and treatment
from your healthcare providers.